Red Yeast Rice

3rd Edition

Rita Elkins, MH

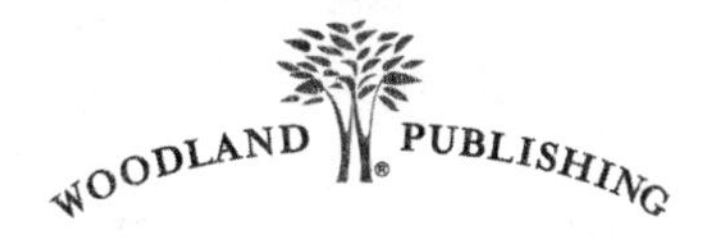

For permissions, ordering information, or bulk quantity discounts, contact:
Woodland Publishing, Salt Lake City, Utah
Visit our website: www.woodlandpublishing.com
Toll-free number: (800) 777-BOOK

The information in this book is for educational purposes only and is not recommended as a means of diagnosing or treating an illness. All matters concerning physical and mental health should be supervised by a health practitioner knowledgeable in treating that particular condition. Neither the publisher nor the author directly or indirectly dispenses medical advice, nor do they prescribe any remedies or assume any responsibility for those who choose to treat themselves.

Cataloging-in-Publication data is available from the Library of Congress.

ISBN: 978-1-58054-200-5

Printed in the United States of America

Contents

Introduction

Nature provides specific compounds that can augment dietary and lifestyle changes and improve cardiovascular health. One of the most impressive of these is a compound extracted from red yeast rice. Red yeast rice is a fermented food substance traditionally used for its red-coloring properties in meats and other foods. In addition to its pigment value, red yeast rice offers some very valuable therapeutic benefits. Red yeast rice has been used throughout Asia for many centuries to lower elevated cholesterol levels.

High cholesterol is a health concern because high levels of cholesterol in the blood increase the risk of cardiovascular disease. According to the American Heart Association (AHA), 35.7 million Americans have abnormally high cholesterol levels, which puts them at a high risk for cardiovascular disease. Another 102.2 million Americans have elevated cholesterol levels that put them at a borderline high risk.

What Is Cholesterol?

In spite of its bad reputation, cholesterol is essential to human life. Cholesterol, a waxy substance found in cell membranes, serves many life-giving functions. Cholesterol is necessary to build healthy cells and synthesize vitamin D for use in the body. The body also needs cholesterol to synthesize important hormones including the sex hormones (progesterone, estrogen and testosterone); cortisol, which the body releases in response to stress; and aldosterone, which helps regulate the body's sodium and potassium levels. Cholesterol is also necessary for the body to manufacture bile salts, which serve an important role in digestion by helping the intestine absorb fat molecules and vitamins that are fat soluble (dissolve in fat), such as vitamins A, D, E and K.

Typically, about 80 percent of the body's cholesterol is manufactured in the body—20 to 25 percent in the liver and the remainder in other tissues and organs. The remaining 20 percent is usually supplied from dietary sources. The body produces less cholesterol when more cholesterol is being supplied from the diet. Dietary cholesterol is found in animal products and byproducts.

What Risks Does High Cholesterol Pose?

With cholesterol, it is possible to have too much of a good thing. While cholesterol in correct amounts is vital, excess cholesterol can collect in the blood. High concentrations of cholesterol in the blood are associated with a few health-threatening complications. Excess cholesterol often clumps in fatty deposits in the blood vessels, leading to two conditions. The first, *atherosclerosis*, occurs when artery walls thicken because of cholesterol deposits. The second, *arteriosclerosis*, happens when the arteries become hardened due to cholesterol buildup. Both of these dangerous conditions can decrease blood flow through the arteries, restricting the amount of blood that gets to tissues and organs, mainly the heart and brain.

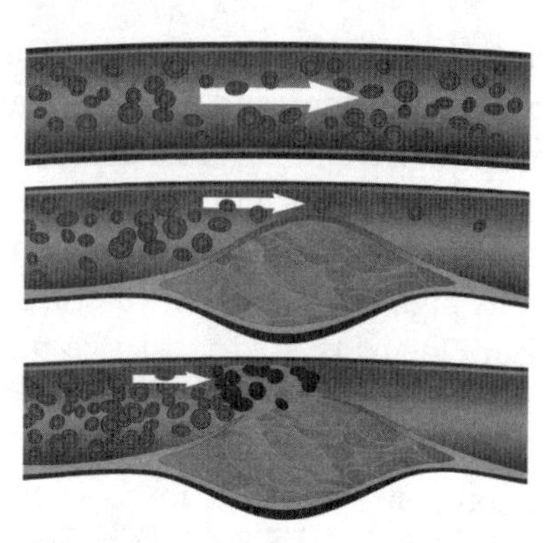

The top artery is healthy, the middle shows the beginning of plaque buildup and the bottom shows plaque blocking off an artery.

Restricting blood flow can be dangerous. Blood carries oxygen, so when blood flow is restricted, the amount of oxygen supplied to tissues and organs also decreases. Partial blockage of arteries can cause chest pain and shortness of breath. Complete blockage can cause a heart attack.

Too much cholesterol can affect other parts of the body as well. An excess of cholesterol can cause bile acids to build up in the gallbladder. A 2007 study in the *Journal of Internal Medicine* reported that when this occurs, the excess bile acids can crystallize, resulting in gallstones.

High cholesterol can be caused by many factors. Cholesterol levels naturally tend to increase with age—partly because the body produces fewer hormones and therefore uses less cholesterol to make them. While aging is not a controllable factor, many other risk factors for developing high cholesterol are controllable. Common risk factors include:

- Obesity
- Inactivity
- Genetic predisposition
- Smoking
- High blood pressure

Poor dietary choices can also cause an increase in blood cholesterol levels. See page 26 for more information on lifestyle and dietary choices that can decrease the risk of developing high cholesterol.

Cholesterol Levels and Coronary Heart Disease

High cholesterol can increase the risk of coronary heart disease (CHD). In someone with CHD, the coronary arteries become blocked or narrowed due to plaque or oxidized cholesterol buildup. Such a buildup can be dangerous to the heart and the brain. Reduced blood flow due to narrowed or blocked arteries can damage the heart. Cholesterol buildup can break off and lodge in the heart or the brain, causing a heart attack or stroke. Major causes of coronary heart disease are similar to risk factors for developing high cholesterol.

CHD is a common disorder in industrialized nations. Many people who die from CHD are otherwise in good health. Like high blood pressure, a related disorder, heart disease can be a silent killer. Symptoms of CHD include impotence, heart attack or stroke.

LDL, HDL and Triglycerides

Healthcare practitioners look at a few indicators in addition to total cholesterol levels to determine risk of heart disease. Three such indicators are high-density lipoprotein (HDL) levels, low-density lipoprotein (LDL) levels and triglyceride levels.

LDL and HDL are not different types of cholesterol. Rather, they are different types of lipoproteins (cholesterol carriers). A lipoprotein is a compound that transports lipids (fats) in the body through the blood. As a lipid, cholesterol can't be dissolved into the blood, so lipoproteins are necessary to transport it through the bloodstream. Lipoproteins are water-soluble on the outside (so they can be dissolved and carried in the blood) while the cholesterol content inside is lipid-soluble.

Both LDL and HDL affect health in dramatically different ways. LDL is the major carrier of cholesterol in the body. It is low density because it contains less protein and more cholesterol. This type of lipoprotein is referred to as "bad cholesterol" because it transports cholesterol from the liver to the bloodstream, predisposing the arteries to plaque buildup and eventual blockage.

HDL is high density because it contains more protein and less cholesterol. It is called "good cholesterol" because it transports cholesterol away from artery walls and back to the liver for storage. This helps prevent cholesterol buildup on artery walls. Higher levels of HDL are usually associated with less atherosclerosis.

A third indicator of heart disease risk is triglyceride level. Triglycerides are another type of lipid found in the blood. The body converts any calories not immediately needed into triglycerides, which are stored in fat cells. Between meals, hormones release triglycerides for the body to use as a quick source of energy. Unlike cholesterol, triglycerides are not necessary for cell building or hormone production. Like cholesterol, high levels of triglycerides in the blood are considered a risk factor for heart disease.

The AHA recommends that everyone over the age of 20 have their cholesterol checked every five years. A cholesterol test analyzes a blood sample taken following a 12-hour fast. A cholesterol test measures total cholesterol levels, HDL levels, LDL levels and triglycerides.

Cholesterol is measured in milligrams per deciliter—a cholesterol level of 200 mg/dL means that there are 200 milligrams of cholesterol in every deciliter of blood. The AHA considers total cholesterol levels of less than 200 mg/dL to be healthy, 200 to 240 mg/dL to be borderline high risk of heart disease and 240 mg/dL or higher to be a high risk for heart disease. Someone with total cholesterol levels above 240 mg/dL or higher has twice the risk of CHD as someone with levels below 200 mg/dL.

For lipoproteins, levels of less than 100 mg/dL of LDL are desirable. Elevated LDL levels are a major risk factor for heart disease. A healthy ratio of total cholesterol to HDL levels in the blood is approximately 5:1. For triglycerides, the AHA recommends that levels should be lower than 150 mg/dL.

Cholesterol By the Numbers

Total Cholesterol Level	Category
Less than 200 mg/dL	Desirable level
200–239 mg/dL	Borderline high cholesterol
240 mg/dL and above	High blood cholesterol

HDL Cholesterol Level	Category
Less than 40 mg/dL (for men) Less than 50 mg/dL (for women)	Unhealthy
60 mg/dL and above	Desirable

LDL Cholesterol Level	Category
Less than 100 mg/dL	Optimal
100–129 mg/dL	Near or above optimal
130–159 mg/dL	Borderline high
160-189 mg/dL	High
190 mg/dL and above	Very high

Triglyceride Level	Category
Less than 150 mg/dL	Normal
150–199 mg/dL	Borderline high
200–499 mg/dL	High
500 mg/dL and above	Very high

Source: *American Heart Association* (www.heart.org)

Treating High Cholesterol

How Statins Work

Improving bad cholesterol levels can be challenging. The body's balance between HDL and LDL is largely determined by genetics. However, this balance can be changed through diet, weight loss and medication or supplementation.

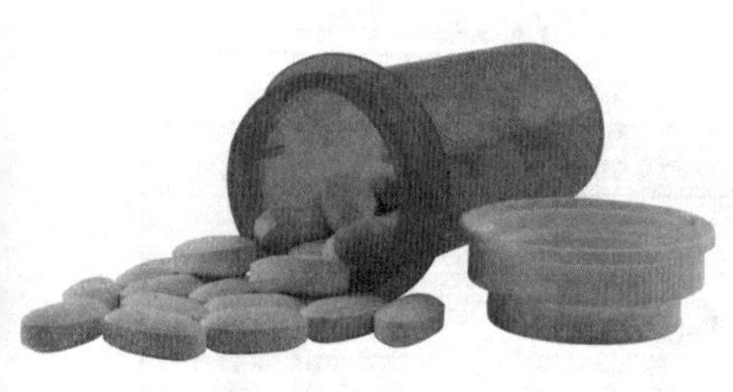

Pharmaceutical medications are commonly prescribed to lower high cholesterol.

Allopathic physicians often prescribe pharmaceutical drugs to lower cholesterol levels. One of the most popular classes of cholesterol-lowering drugs is *statins*, including Lipitor®, Crestor®, Mevacor® (lovastatin) and Zocor®. Red yeast rice also contains a small amount of a naturally-occurring statin called monacolin K. See page 13 for differences and similarities between red yeast rice and statin drugs.

In 2010, statins were some of the most profitable prescription drugs in America, according to IMS Health, a company that provides market information about pharmaceutical companies. Statins lower cholesterol by slowing the body's cholesterol production. Statins inhibit production of 3-hydroxy-3-methylglutaryl coenzyme A reductase (HMG-CoA reductase), an enzyme required in a key step of cholesterol synthesis. When HMG-CoA reductase is inhibited, the body's production of cholesterol is slowed. Statins can also stabilize atherosclerotic plaque in the coronary arteries, decreasing the risk of complications due to artery blockage. Other studies show that statins change lipoprotein patterns from unhealthy to healthy by increasing HDL and decreasing LDL. The overall effect is a decrease in cardiovascular disease risk.

Discovery of Statins

Initially, HMG-CoA reductase inhibitors were discovered by accident. Researchers discovered certain compounds that lowered cholesterol while researching antifungal agents. Unfortunately, the compounds initially discovered were also highly toxic; therefore, their ability to decrease cholesterol was not applicable. The idea of discovering another metabolite that could treat high cholesterol by blocking the action of HMG-CoA reductase without toxicity motivated further research.

A breakthrough came in 1980. Scientists in New Jersey isolated lovastatin from a fungal strain of *Aspergillus terreus*, a fungus commonly used to produce organic acids. This compound was later introduced as the first HMG-CoA reductase inhibitor, lovastatin. Naturally-occurring lovastatin is found in oyster mushrooms. Scientists isolate and condense the compound to synthesize pharmaceutical drugs.

The success of lovastatin prompted research to find other methods of inhibiting HMG-CoA reductase. At the same time, other chemical compounds were derived from lovastatin in an attempt to synthesize a superior product. In synthetically produced statins, scientists examine plant chemistry, isolate what they consider the most active compound and then artificially reproduce it.

Cholesterol-lowering pharmaceutical drugs have pros and cons. Artificially refining or synthesizing various compounds into high doses in order to create a pharmaceutical drug can lead to toxicity. When a medicinal ingredient occurs in a natural compound, it is found in combination with other natural ingredients. Natural compounds work in tandem with the body's natural processes, thereby avoiding many (but not always all) detrimental side effects associated with prescription medication. Frequently, when the active principle of an herbal medicine is isolated, such as the monacolin K from red yeast rice, the synergistic balancing effect of the entire herb is lost. In other words, artificial compounds may offer valuable therapeutic benefits, but they may cause a number of unwanted reactions as well. Prescription drugs can be lifesavers, but check with a healthcare practitioner to determine all possible courses of action.

Pharmaceutical drugs also commonly have noted side effects. Drugs created from isolated or synthetic compounds may be more potent and easier to ingest; however, the human body tends to recognize them as foreign and unnatural substances. This may result in a chain of physiological reactions, characterized by adverse effects. Even in prescription drugs that use compounds isolated from natural sources, the medicinal compound is synthesized in a way that makes side effects more potent as well. Frequently, such a purified and concentrated chemical may overwhelm certain metabolic activities or enzymes, competing with other nutrients or depressing certain systems, causing side effects.

Many people who take pharmaceutical statins experience side effects. Common side effects associated with statins include headache, dizziness, rash and upset stomach. Less commonly, taking statins can result in *myalgia*, or muscle pain. A related and more serious side effect is *myopathy*, a muscular disease where muscles do not function properly, resulting in muscle weakness, cramps, stiffness or spasm. Statins are also sometimes associated with liver damage. The risk of these potentially serious side effects is one reason that statin drugs are offered by prescription instead of over-the-counter (OTC).

Red Yeast Rice

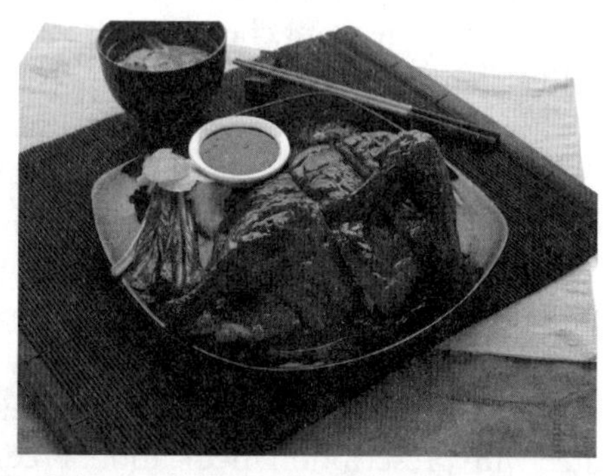

Red yeast rice has traditionally been used to give Peking duck its red hue.

Red yeast rice is derived from *Monascus purpureus*, a rice that is fermented by the addition of yeast. It is also called *hong qu*. It is a deep crimson color and has been used for centuries to give foods a rich, stable red color. In traditional Chinese cooking, red yeast rice is used to color Peking duck, cha siu bao (pork buns), cheese and rice wine. The advantage of using red yeast rice to color food is that it is considered nontoxic and remains stable even when exposed to high temperatures. However, synthetic dyes are widely available, so many cooks now use red dye instead of red yeast rice to achieve a red color.

During the Ming Dynasty (between 1368 and 1644 AD), red yeast rice was described as "sweet in flavor and warm in property" by noted pharmocologist of the time, Li Shizhen. It has been commonly used in the Fujian region on the southeast coast of China for thousands of years to enhance the flavor of foods. In this region, people typically consume between 14 and 55 grams of red yeast daily, sprinkling it on main dishes like tofu as a colorful topping.

Traditional Medicinal Uses

Red yeast rice is more than just a food dye and topping. In addition to its culinary uses, red yeast rice also has medicinal value.

Red yeast rice has long been used in Chinese medicine. The earliest documented use of red yeast rice is during the Tang Dynasty in 800 AD. It is mentioned in a traditional Chinese pharmacopoeia (a book containing descriptions of medicinal compounds) published during the Ming Dynasty. In this pharmacopoeia, red yeast rice is suggested as a treatment for mild gastric problems (including indigestion and diarrhea), to promote blood circulation and for stomach and spleen health. Red yeast rice has also been traditionally used as a treatment for dysentery, to reduce swelling, to treat wounds and cuts and as a treatment for cancer. Scientific studies for these uses are limited.

Red Yeast Rice for Cholesterol

In 1976, Japanese scientist Dr. Akira Endo isolated a metabolite of red yeast rice called monacolin K (from the word *Monascus*). As Endo and other researchers began to experiment with monacolin K, they discovered that it significantly reduced artifically-induced high cholesterol levels in laboratory test rats. Their research indicated that monacolin K, like pharmaceutical statins, inhibits HMG-CoA reductase.

Red yeast rice supplements may be helpful for individuals who suffer from moderately high cholesterol levels. Supplements can be incorporated into an overall therapeutic strategy that includes diet and exercise. Red yeast rice supplements should not be viewed as a cure for any condition, but rather as one of the natural ways to help support desirable cholesterol levels.

Scientific Validation of Red Yeast Rice

The Wang Study

The first human study of red yeast rice was conducted in China in 1997. A team of researchers led by Junxian Wang studied 446 patients who were diagnosed with high cholesterol and triglyceride levels. All test subjects had total cholesterol levels of 230 mg/dL or higher and an LDL count higher than 130 mg/dL. In addition, the patients had an HDL count of less than or equal to 40 mg/dL for men and 45 mg/dL for women. Anyone who had suffered from a heart attack, stroke, major surgery or diabetes within the previous six months was not allowed to participate in the study.

Patients were randomly divided into two groups. The 324 patients in the treatment group were given 600 mg of red yeast rice twice a day (1200 mg/day) and the patients in the control group were given a Chinese herb called *Jiaogulan*, also reputed to have cholesterol-lowering properties. Cholesterol levels were measured before the start of the study and at the ends of weeks four and eight. After four weeks of therapy with red yeast rice, total cholesterol levels decreased by 17.1 percent compared to a reduction of 4.8 percent in the control group. LDL count in the red yeast rice group was reduced by an average of 24.6 percent versus an average of 6.3 percent in the control group. Serum triglycerides decreased by an average of 19.8 percent in the treatment group and 9.2 percent in the control group. In addition, HDL levels increased by 12.8 percent with red yeast rice and 4.9 percent without.

At the end of eight weeks of treatment, the patients in the treatment group had an average reduction in total cholesterol of 22.7 percent versus an average reduction of 7 percent in the control group. *Red yeast rice supplementation had reduced their LDL levels by* ***30.9*** *percent.* This reduction was significantly greater than that in the control group. Total blood triglyceride levels were reduced by 34.1 percent with red yeast rice and 12.8 percent without. Adverse reactions to red yeast rice were rare and fairly mild—six people experienced heartburn, three experienced "flatulence in the stomach" and one experienced dizziness.

Researchers concluded that red yeast rice is a "highly effective and well tolerated dietary supplement that can be used to regulate elevated serum cholesterol and triglycerides."

Other Studies

American researchers have also discovered the benefits of red yeast rice. The first American study on red yeast rice was conducted two years later at the University of California, Los Angeles (UCLA) and supports the idea that red yeast rice can lower cholesterol far more than just dietary or exercise changes. This double-blind, randomized study was published in 1999 in the *American Journal of Clinical*

Nutrition. It examined the cholesterol-lowering effects of red yeast rice in patients with moderately high to high cholesterol levels (204 to 338 mg/dL) and LDL levels between 128 and 277 mg/dL. At the time of the study, none of the patients were being treated with lipid lowering drugs.

The study examined diet and lifestyle in addition to supplementation. All 83 subjects were given a pamphlet detailing the AHA's dietary recommendations. The pamphlet recommends consuming less than 30 percent of energy from fat, less than 10 percent from saturated fat and less than 300 mg of cholesterol daily. The subjects were randomized into either the red yeast rice group or the placebo group. Those in the red yeast rice group received a capsule containing 2400 mg of red yeast rice daily, while the placebo group received a similar-looking capsule.

As in the Wang study, red yeast rice significantly lowered cholesterol levels. Researchers took blood samples before the beginning of the study, after eight weeks and after 12 weeks. After eight weeks, the total cholesterol of every member of the red yeast rice group had decreased, while there was no significant difference in total cholesterol concentration of the placebo group. Cholesterol levels decreased further when measured at the 12-week mark.

Red yeast rice also lowered LDL levels. LDL levels decreased in the group treated with red yeast rice, but not in the placebo group. Unlike the Wang study, researchers in this study found no significant change in HDL levels. The researchers concluded that red yeast rice reduced cholesterol concentrations more than diet alone, without significant adverse effects.

RYR as a Statin Substitute

Many people are reluctant to take pharmaceutical statins. Doctors recommend that people who begin taking statins should continue to do so indefinitely unless directed otherwise by a healthcare practitioner. Many people disregard this advice. As much as 40 percent of individuals who receive prescriptions for statins take them for less than one year. Doctors attribute this to several factors, including cost, lack of understanding of statin benefits, reluctance to take prescription medications long term and side effects associated with pharmaceutical statins.

Muscle pain is one of the biggest reasons individuals stop taking pharmaceutical statins. Red yeast rice may be a good alternative to pharmaceutical statins for such individuals. Because the monacolin K in red yeast rice occurs in naturally low doses, it is generally better tolerated in the body.

One recent study supports this theory. In a 2009 study published in the *Annals of Internal Medicine*, researchers looked at red yeast rice as an alternative for patients who could not take statins due to muscle pain. This study looked at 62 patients with high cholesterol who had previously stopped using pharmaceutical statins because of muscle pain. Patients were randomly assigned to receive either a placebo or 1800 mg of red yeast rice daily for 24 weeks. In addition, all participants were enrolled in a 12-week program intended to improve dietary and exercise habits.

In this study, red yeast rice lowered cholesterol without causing muscle pain. After the 24-week trial period, LDL levels had decreased an average of 35 mg/dL in members of the red yeast rice group, significantly more than members of the placebo group. Total cholesterol levels also improved more in the red yeast rice group than in the placebo group. More importantly for this study, researchers found no difference in muscle pain between the two groups. The researchers concluded that red yeast rice was a potential way for patients who can't tolerate pharmaceutical statins to lower cholesterol levels.

Active Ingredients

As a naturally-occurring substance, red yeast rice has no single "active ingredient." It contains multiple compounds that may contribute to its medicinal properties. Different strains of red yeast rice can also contain different concentrations of various compounds.

Initially, scientists attributed red yeast rice's ability to lower cholesterol entirely to the presence of a lovastatin-like compound called monacolin K. However, subsequent research found that red yeast rice contains much smaller amounts of monacolin K than is typically considered an effective dose, yet red yeast rice continues to have cholesterol-lowering effects. In the studies discussed previously, the average dosage of red yeast rice was 1200 to 2400 mg per day. Such a dose contains about 10 mg of monacolins on average, about half of which are monacolin K. The dose of statins typically considered effective is 20 to 28 mg per day. Hence, scientists continue to study other components of red yeast rice to determine how they work together with monacolin K to produce cholesterol-lowering effects.

Monacolin K is not the only compound found in red yeast rice. Red yeast rice contains many other monacolins, including monacolin X and dihydromonacolin L, both of which are structurally related to monacolin K. In addition, red yeast rice contains monacolin J, L, M and X and dihydromonacolin K, which are precursors to monacolin K. These compounds are not well understood. Some may have lipid-lowering qualities, or they may enhance the lipid-lowering properties of monacolin K. Regardless, the monacolins in red yeast rice work together to enhance the cholesterol-lowering capability of the substance.

Red yeast rice contains more than monacolins. It also contains a variety of other compounds with cholesterol-lowering capabilities. Red yeast rice contains both monounsaturated and polyunsaturated fatty acids. In other substances, mono and polyunsaturated fatty acids have been found to increase levels of HDL and decrease LDL levels. The presence of such "healthy fats" in red yeast rice may also increase the body's ability to clear cholesterol.

Another substance found in red yeast rice is a class of plant compounds called *phytosterols*. Phytosterols are the plant equivalent of cholesterol and are found in all plants. In a 2007 study published in *Lipids*, researchers reported that phytosterols can reduce the body's cholesterol absorption. Phytosterols bind to receptor sites, preventing cholesterol from being absorbed into the bloodstream through the intestinal wall. The overall result is that more cholesterol is eliminated from the body. Phytosterols found in red yeast rice include beta-sitosterol, campesterol, stigmasterol and sapogenin.

The fiber content of red yeast rice may also contribute to its medicinal effect. For more information on how fiber can help reduce cholesterol levels, see page 29.

Safety Issues

Many researchers consider red yeast rice to be safe. After all, it has been used in Chinese cuisine and medicine for centuries. However, while isolation and concentration to increase potency is the main cause of side effects with pharmaceutical statins, red yeast rice supplements may also cause some side effects in susceptible individuals.

Adverse effects may include heartburn, upset stomach and dizziness.

As with any dietary supplement regimen, use red yeast rice supplements under the supervision of a healthcare practitioner. Check cholesterol levels after a two-month course of therapy. As mentioned, statins are sometimes linked with liver damage. Researchers also recommend asking a healthcare practitioner to monitor liver function to make sure that red yeast rice does not cause adverse effects to the liver.

Some people should avoid red yeast rice. Since cholesterol is an essential component of cell membranes, it is vital for proper fetal and infant development. Therefore, women who are pregnant or breastfeeding should avoid red yeast rice supplements (and other statins). Children should *not* take this supplement unless advised to do so by a healthcare practitioner.

Anyone currently taking prescription drugs to control cholesterol levels should not take red yeast rice without the approval of a healthcare practitioner. Those who are currently taking cholesterol-lowering prescription drugs should not stop taking them or alter dosage in any way without consulting a healthcare practitioner. Those with allergies to yeast or fungus should avoid red yeast rice, as should anyone with kidney or liver disease or infection.

Be wary of red yeast products that contain high amounts of monacolins. Although the monacolin content of red yeast rice supplements can vary from one brand to another or even batch to batch, some companies may "spike" red yeast rice supplements by adding extra monacolin K. Higher than normal content may lead to the same complications associated with pharmaceutical statins.

Further, avoid grapefruit and grapefruit juice while taking red yeast rice supplements. Grapefruit can slow how quickly the body uses red yeast rice, increasing the chance of side effects. Do not drink more than two alcoholic drinks per day if taking red yeast rice due to potential liver damage.

Finally, some brands of red yeast rice supplements may be contaminated with citrinin, a fungal toxin. This is a concern as animal testing has shown that citrinin may cause kidney failure. It is unclear whether citrinin affects humans. To avoid this danger, choose a reputable brand of red yeast rice that screens its products for citrinin.

Red Yeast Rice and the FDA

Is red yeast rice a drug or a nutritional supplement? This question has been at the center of a legal dispute since 1998. Some argue that the monacolin K in red yeast rice is structurally identical to lovastatin, and therefore red yeast rice is subject to regulation as a pharmaceutical drug.

In the United States, the Food and Drug Administration (FDA) regulates dietary supplements differently than prescription and OTC medications. All dietary supplements, including red yeast rice, are regulated under the Dietary Supplement Health and Education Act of 1994 (DSHEA), an amendment to the Federal Food, Drug and Cosmetic Act of 1938.

Under this act, supplement manufacturers are responsible for testing their products for safety, and for making sure that label information is accurate and not misleading. If the FDA suspects a product is unsafe or a label is misleading, the administration takes action.

The FDA also regulates ingredients of dietary supplements. Under DSHEA, any product that is sold as a "dietary supplement" can't contain ingredients that have been approved as ingredients in new drugs, unless the supplement was marketed before the drug's approval.

In 1998, the FDA began action to ban Cholestin®, which at the time was the product name of a supplement containing red yeast rice. In May 1998, the FDA ruled that Cholestin® should be considered an unapproved new drug, not a dietary supplement. Although Pharmanex, Inc., the company that produced Cholestin®, argued that monacolin is similar but not identical to lovastatin, a U.S. District Court upheld the original ruling. The FDA asked Pharmanex to reformulate Cholestin® to remove its red yeast rice content and restricted the sale of red yeast rice. Because of the potentially dangerous side effects of pharmaceutical statins, the FDA viewed the unregulated sale of powerful statin medications as dietary supplements as dangerous.

Following this ruling, products containing red yeast rice disappeared from the market for a short time. They began to reappear in 2003 after being reformulated to include only naturally-produced red yeast rice. By 2010 there were approximately 30 brands available.

Red yeast rice products currently on the market make no claims to contain monacolin or lower cholesterol, in line with DSHEA. All of these products are fermented according to traditional Asian methods, to ensure that they have the naturally-occurring benefits of red yeast rice without the side effects associated with high monacolin K levels.

Other Potential Benefits of Red Yeast Rice

Red yeast rice may have other benefits as well. While cholesterol-lowering is the best-known and most widely studied benefit of red yeast rice, it has been studied for other applications. In connection with its cholesterol benefits, researchers have studied the use of red yeast rice to treat heart disease. Limited scientific studies suggest that red yeast rice may also have anti-cancer effects and benefits for diabetes.

Red Yeast Rice and Heart Disease

High cholesterol is not the only factor that leads to heart disease. Research suggests that inflammation is also a huge factor. Red yeast rice may fight heart disease by not only decreasing the amount of cholesterol in the body but also by fighting inflammation. The AHA suggests that measuring levels of C-reactive protein, a protein that increases in the blood when inflammation is present, may be one way to measure risk of heart disease. Inflammation makes high cholesterol worse because it encourages cholesterol to bind to places it shouldn't, such as arterial walls. A study published in 2004 in *Circulation*, the journal of the AHA, reported that in clinical trials, red yeast rice decreased levels of C-reactive protein.

Red yeast rice may lower the risk of heart attack and stroke. In 2007, a study published in the *Journal of Cardiovascular Pharmacology* looked at the effect of red yeast rice in patients with CHD. The study examined 591 patients with diabetes and 4279 patients without diabetes. Subjects were randomly divided into a red yeast rice group or a placebo group. The red yeast rice group took 600 mg of red yeast rice twice daily. The study tracked these individuals for an average of four years and found that in the diabetes group taking red yeast rice, risk for a CHD event (chest pain, heart attack, stroke, heart failure, etc.) was reduced 50.8

percent. Risk for a CHD event in those without diabetes taking red yeast rice was reduced 43.9 percent. This study also found that red yeast rice reduced C-reactive protein levels and improved blood vessel widening. The researchers suggested that these effects may be the reason red yeast rice helps decrease heart disease risk.

Red Yeast Rice and Tumors

Red yeast rice has been studied for years for potential cancer-inhibiting properties. Research about the use of red yeast rice to inhibit tumor growth is ongoing, but it suggests that red yeast rice is a potential botanical means of preventing the growth of tumor cells.

Early research focused on red yeast rice pigment. A clinical study, published in *Oncology* in 1996, was conducted at the College of Pharmacy of Nihon University in Japan. Researchers found that red yeast rice pigment, referred to as *Monascus* pigment, was able to inhibit the growth of malignant tumors induced in laboratory test mice. These scientists extracted the *Monascus* pigment from red yeast rice and administered it orally.

Other studies have focused on monacolin K as the anti-cancer agent in red yeast rice. Studies demonstrate that individuals taking statins have a decreased risk of colon cancer. Cholesterol synthesis is required for tumor growth, so inhibiting cholesterol synthesis may help inhibit cancer cell growth. A 2007 study published in the *Journal of Agriculture and Food Chemistry* found that by inhibiting HMG-CoA reductase, monacolin K also suppressed the growth of cancer cells.

Red yeast rice is a complex compound. A study published in 2008 in the *Journal of Nutritional Biochemistry* recognized the complexity of red yeast rice and examined the combined anti-cancer effects of the *Monascus* pigment and monacolin K. The researchers purified red yeast rice to be pigment-rich or monacolin-rich and tested the effects of these different strains on human colon cancer cells. The researchers found that the monacolin-rich strain decreased cell growth and induced apoptosis (cell death). The pigment-rich strain also inhibited cell growth and enhanced apoptosis. The researchers concluded that the anti-cancer effects of red yeast rice were due to more than just monacolin K content. Multiple components of red yeast rice may play a role in its potential cancer-inhibiting ability.

Red Rice and Diabetes

Red yeast rice may also help treat diabetes. Preliminary studies suggest that red yeast rice has benefits for diabetes, although further studies in humans are necessary to confirm action. A study conducted in 2006 and published in *Neuroscience Letters* reported that red yeast rice (called hon-chi in the study) decreased blood sugar and increased insulin levels in rats. The researchers suggested that red yeast rice helps stimulate pancreatic cells, increasing insulin release.

Complementary Supplements

Many other supplements can work in conjunction with red yeast rice supplements to control cholesterol levels. Consult a healthcare practitioner prior to beginning any dietary supplement regimen.

Coenzyme Q10

Coenzyme Q10 (CoQ10) is a compound found at the center of cells that is involved in energy production. It is vital to the healthy functioning of the body, especially the immune and cardiovascular systems. Production of this enzyme tends to decrease with age, and studies have found that people with high levels of cholesterol often have lower levels of CoQ10. A deficiency of CoQ10 is associated with cardiovascular disease.

As previously discussed, statins lower cholesterol production by inhibiting the body's production of HMG-CoA reductase. However, this does not only affect HMG-CoA reductase. Statins also inhibit production of CoQ10. This means that those taking both natural and synthetic statins should consider CoQ10 supplementation to make up for any deficiency statin therapy may cause.

On its own, CoQ10 supplements may effectively lower heart disease risk. CoQ10 may help treat congestive heart failure, a condition where the heart does not pump blood effectively, and may cause blood to pool in the lungs and legs. According to the *Natural Standard*, an online database that provides information about complementary and alternative medicine, CoQ10 is routinely used as part of therapy for congestive heart failure in Europe, Russia and Japan.

A study published in 2009 in *Pharmacology and Therapeutics* found that CoQ10 inhibits LDL oxidation and decreases inflammation. The study also found that CoQ10 decreases the viscosity of blood. Blood viscosity measures how thick the blood is, and hence how resistant it is to flowing through the veins. Thicker or more viscous blood causes the heart to work harder, decreasing the amount of oxygen delivered to the brain, heart and tissues. In addition, the study found that CoQ10 supplementation may be helpful for individuals who experience muscle pain due to statin therapy.

Essential Fatty Acids

Although some people think that all fats contribute to high cholesterol, essential fatty acids (EFAs) are vital to every living cell in the body. EFAs are divided into different categories, including omega-3s and omega-6s, depending on their chemical structure. Both omega-3 and omega-6 fatty acids can help decrease blood pressure and blood lipids. Omega-3 fatty acids may also fight inflammation and protect the brain and nervous system. Omega-3s are found in fresh deepwater fish such as tuna, anchovy, sardine, mackerel and salmon as well as certain vegetable oils including flaxseed oil, canola oil and walnut oil. Omega-6 fatty acids are found in raw nuts, especially walnuts, seeds including hemp and pumpkin and vegetable oils such as borage oil, black currant oil, grape seed oil, evening primrose oil and sesame oil.

A 2008 study published in *Mayo Clinic Proceedings* examined the effect of fish oil and red yeast rice as part of a potential treatment option for patients with high blood cholesterol. Seventy-four subjects who met standard criteria for taking pharmaceutical statins participated. The participants were then divided into either a statin group or an alternative treatment group. Both groups received treatment for three months. The statin group received 40 mg of a pharmaceutical statin daily and read printed materials about diet and exercise recommendations (the standard allopathic treatment for high cholesterol). The alternative treatment group received daily fish oil and red yeast rice supplements and attended weekly 3.5 hour education meetings taught by a dietitian, cardiologist, exercise physiologist and several alternative practitioners.

The study found that the fish oil and red yeast rice group experienced lower cholesterol levels. Both groups experienced a reduction of LDL cholesterol—about 39.6 percent for the statin group and 42.4

percent for the alternative treatment group. Members of the "alternative" group who received both red yeast rice and fish oil supplements also lost more weight and experienced a substantial reduction of triglycerides.

Other Helpful Supplements

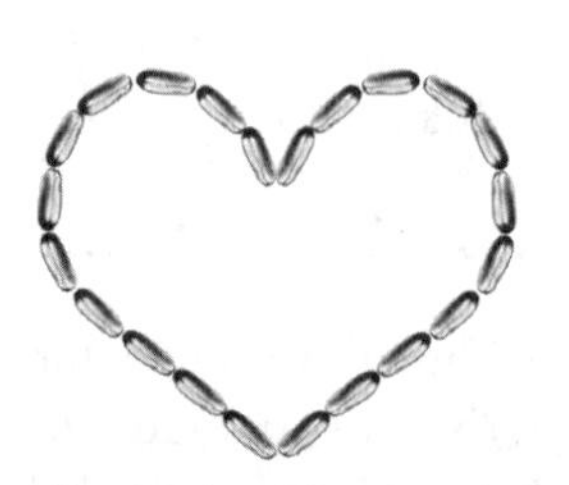

Diet, exercise and nutritional supplemetns can protect the health of the heart.

B-Vitamins. B-complex vitamins, particularly B_6, B_{12} and folic acid, can be important in helping elevated cholesterol levels. Such vitamins are required to break down *homocysteine*, an amino acid that at elevated levels is associated with an increased risk of atherosclerosis, heart attack, stroke and blood clot formation.

Chitosan. Chitosan is derived from a substance found in the shells of crustaceans such as shrimp, crab or lobster and also in mushrooms and yeasts. Farmers use chitosan as a natural seed growth enhancer and in water purification to absorb grease, metal and oil. In a 2003 study published in the *European Journal of Clinical Nutrition* researchers gave 1200 mg of chitosan daily to subjects with moderately high cholesterol who made no alterations to their diets. The researchers found that chitosan had a mild effect of lowering total cholesterol and LDL levels. Why? Because it binds to dietary fats and cholesterol in the intestines, preventing their absorption.

Chromium. Chromium is a mineral that the body needs in trace amounts. It assists in the metabolism of carbohydrates, fats and proteins. Studies suggest that chromium supplementation may help raise HDL levels. The recommended dosage is about 500 mcg daily.

Garlic. Garlic (*Allium sativum*), an herb from the onion family, has been used for medicinal as well as culinary purposes throughout the world for thousands of years. Numerous studies support the effectiveness of garlic in lowering blood cholesterol levels, as detailed in a review of herbal treatments for high blood cholesterol published in 2007 in *Alternative Therapies in Health and Medicine*. The recommended dosage is 500 to 1000 mg in a pure powdered extract. Odorless and tasteless forms of garlic are available.

Ginger. The root of the ginger (*Zingiber officinale*) plant has been used medicinally in China and India for centuries. Ginger is widely used as a treatment for nausea, but studies suggest that it can reduce cholesterol levels by inhibiting its absorption. Further study is needed, but a study published in 2008 in the *Saudi Medical Journal* found that a dose of one gram of ginger three times daily reduced cholesterol, triglyceride and LDL levels. Ginger increases bile flow, which is important for breaking down cholesterol.

When taken in large quantities, ginger can cause stomach discomfort. The maximum recommended dose of ginger is four grams daily. People who take anticoagulants should avoid ginger due to an increased risk of bleeding problems. People with gallstones may experience pain when taking ginger because it constricts the bowel ducts, potentially squeezing any gallstones inside the bowel ducts.

Guggul. Guggul comes from the sap of the mukul myrrh tree, which is native to India. Guggul has been used in traditional ayurvedic medicine for centuries—an ayurvedic text from 600 BC recommends using guggul to treat atherosclerosis. Currently, an extract of guggul called gugulipid is used to treat high cholesterol and atherosclerosis. Studies suggest that gugulipid helps in the production of bile and also prevents blood platelets from clumping together, helping to prevent atherosclerosis.

Lecithin. Every cell in the body needs lecithin. It is made mostly of choline, a B-vitamin. Although lecithin is a lipid it is partly water-soluble and helps remove other lipids, such as cholesterol, from the body. This protects the body against arteriosclerosis.

A 2003 study published in the *Journal of the American Dietetic Association* examined how effectively lecithin reduced high LDL and cholesterol levels. Subjects of the study consumed a lemonade-flavored drink containing lecithin powder daily for four weeks. The researchers found that lecithin reduced cholesterol absorption, reducing both total cholesterol and LDL levels.

Niacin. The AHA includes niacin (vitamin B_3) in its recommendations for a "first line" treatment of elevated cholesterol. This B-vitamin is necessary for proper blood circulation. Niacin (not niacinamide) supplements may help to lower LDL levels, increase HDL levels and improve the total cholesterol to HDL ratio. A 1995 study published in the *American Journal of Cardiology* found that taking niacin and lovastatin together improved cholesterol more significantly than either substance alone. Do not take high doses (more than 500 mg daily) as it can harm the liver. Niacin briefly causes flushing and itching at elevated levels. For a non-flushing version, try inositol hexanicotinate.

Policosanol. Policosanol is a mixture of fatty alcohols derived from sugar cane, yams and beeswax. It is used to lower LDL levels and increase HDL levels. Studies have shown that it can inhibit blood platelet clumping and help lower cholesterol. Generally, a dosage of between five to 40 grams daily is considered safe.

Vitamin E. Vitamin E is a powerful antioxidant, a substance that neutralizes the damaging effects of compounds called *free radicals*. A free radical is an atom that is unstable because it lacks an electron. Free radicals take electrons from other atoms, creating more free radicals in a continuous chain. This process, called oxidation, damages cells and can increase the risk of heart disease. Oxidized LDL is a factor in increasing risk of heart disease, and vitamin E helps prevent this oxidation. Vitamin E may also help prevent blood clots. A dose of about 400 IU daily is considered safe and effective.

Other Cholesterol Management Guidelines

Lifestyle changes can be an important addition to supplements such as red yeast rice when trying to lower cholesterol. Many of the studies mentioned include dietary and lifestyle changes along with red yeast rice supplementation. Dietary changes, exercise and stress management can all play a role in cholesterol management.

Dietary Guidelines

Fats

Previously, nutritionists taught that all fats were unhealthy, but recent research contradicts that premise. The body needs fat—it helps the nervous system function properly and is necessary for the body to absorb certain vitamins. Fat is also important to maintaining healthy hair and skin. However, there are different types of fat, and some are healthier than others.

First, the fats to avoid. Saturated fat and trans fat deserve the bad reputation associated with fats. Saturated fats are associated with clogged arteries, high LDL levels and elevated total cholesterol. This type of fat is solid at room temperature. Animal products tend to contain higher amounts of saturated fat, so limit red meat, butter, sour cream and whole-fat dairy products including cheese and milk.

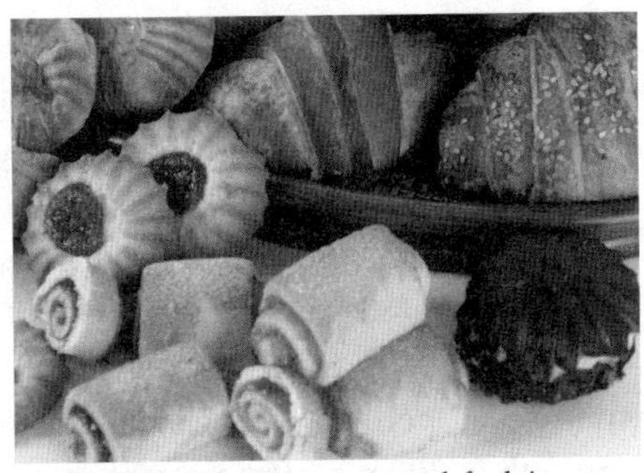

Trans fats are found in many snack foods in addition to fried and fast food.

There are a few exceptions to this rule. Saturated fat found in fruits and vegetables can be beneficial. And coconut oil, a saturated fat, is possibly the healthiest option for cooking and baking.

The most harmful type of fat is trans fat. Trans fats are created when a liquid vegetable oil is hydrogenated (converted) to make a solid fat. Such fats are considered particularly unhealthy because they not only raise LDL and total cholesterol levels but also lower HDL levels. Many people associate trans fats with fried foods, but they are also commonly found in cookies, cakes, pies, pastries and snack foods.

Unsaturated fat is considered "good" fat. Unsaturated fat can help fight diseases, including heart disease, stroke and diabetes. This type of fat can benefit cholesterol levels when used in place of saturated fat. A study conducted in 2010 at Harvard University and published in the *Public Library of Science Medicine* found that replacing saturated fats with an equal amount of unsaturated fat lowered the risk of heart disease by 19 percent.

There are two types of unsaturated fat: monounsaturated and polyunsaturated. Monounsaturated fats can be helpful in lowering LDL and raising HDL levels. Polyunsaturated fats are a good source of omega-3 essential fatty acids. (Benefits of omega-3 are discussed on page 23.) No food source contains only one or the other, but good sources of monounsaturated fat include olive oil, canola oil and avocados. Good sources of polyunsaturated fat include dark leafy green vegetables such as kale, spinach and mustard greens, flaxseed and flaxseed oil and coldwater fish.

A few simple changes can reduce unhealthy hydrogenated and trans fats in the diet. Avoid processed foods and use liquid oils such as olive oil and coconut oil in place of solid fats in cooking and baking. Eat more fish (especially wild salmon) and soy foods such as tofu. Choose lean cuts of meat and low-fat dairy products.

Even "good" fats are still fats and can be harmful to health if consumed in excess. There is no such thing as a "light" or "low-fat" oil. Unsaturated fats still contain a lot of calories. The United States Department of Agriculture (USDA) recommends consuming less than seven percent of one's daily calories from animal fats, and no more than 200 mg of cholesterol per day. To lower high cholesterol, limit consumption of the following foods:

- Beef
- Egg yolks
- Fast food
- Shellfish
- White flour
- White sugar

Completely eliminating certain foods may not be as important as balancing them or using them in moderation. Ancel Keys, a scientist who studied the effect of diets on health, made groundbreaking discoveries in what is now called the "Mediterranean diet." He observed a much higher content of plasma cholesterol in men from Minnesota as compared to men from Naples, Italy that could not be explained by their patterns of fatty acid or cholesterol intake. His study indicated that the Italians ate foods higher in saturated fats such as butter and meat but also large amounts of grains, vegetables, legumes and fruits, which seemed to control cholesterol levels. Keys' findings suggest that controlling high cholesterol is much more complicated than simply eliminating saturated fats.

Naturally, if suffering from elevated cholesterol, it is important to limit consumption of animal fats. It is also true, however, that using the right supplements and foods together helps to balance and control cholesterol.

The Fiber Component

Fiber doesn't just help digestion. Boosting soluble fiber intake can be one of the most effective treatments for high blood cholesterol levels when combined with dietary changes and other natural components.

There are two types of fiber—soluble and insoluble. Insoluble fiber benefits bowel function—it is indigestible and passes through the digestive system in its original form. This increases the bulk of the stool and helps other food material move through the digestive system, improving bowel function. Soluble fiber dissolves in water, forming a gel that traps fat and slows the body's absorption of sugar. Because it forms this gel, soluble fiber stays in the stomach longer, slowing food absorption.

The AHA recommends eating foods that are high in both kinds of fiber, although soluble fiber is the most beneficial to lowering blood cholesterol levels. Soluble fiber helps lower cholesterol in several ways. First, this type of fiber binds with dietary fats, bile and cholesterol found in the intestines. This means that less cholesterol and bile are returned to the bloodstream through the intestines, which lowers cholesterol levels. Soluble fiber also influences the secretion of insulin, which affects how lipids are broken down in the bloodstream and stored.

Plant-based foods are the best sources of soluble fiber. Soluble fiber-rich foods include:

- Barley
- Beans
- Bran
- Oatmeal
- Peas
- Rice

Numerous studies support the use of soluble fiber in lowering cholesterol. A 2008 study published in *Current Atherosclerosis Reports* reported that dietary fiber, particularly soluble fiber, helped to lower LDL cholesterol levels, decreasing the risk of cardiovascular disease. In addition, psyllium has also proven to be a cholesterol inhibitor.

Note: Do not take any fiber supplement at the same time you take other nutrient supplements to avoid any interference with fat-soluble vitamins, etc.

Exercise

Exercise is also an integral component to maintaining good cardiovascular health. The AHA notes that aerobic exercise is beneficial to the heart and recommends getting 150 minutes of moderate exercise each week. That breaks down to approximately 30 minutes of exercise each day, which is equally beneficial when broken into two or three 10 to 15 minute segments.

The AHA particularly recommends walking as the single most effective way to achieve heart health. According to AHA data, life expectancy increases two hours for every hour spent walking. Implement an exercise regimen under the guidelines set by a healthcare practitioner.

Stress and Cholesterol Levels

Chronic and poorly-managed stress can affect cholesterol levels by increasing inflammation. Learning to deal with stress is important in controlling high blood pressure and high cholesterol. When the body is under stress, the brain signals the release of hormones such as adrenaline and cortisol. Both of these hormones trigger the production of cholesterol, which can increase cholesterol levels in the body. Cortisol also raises blood sugar, and the body converts unused sugar to triglycerides, further increasing the risk of heart disease.

Unmanaged stress can contribute to plaque formation and obstruction. Learning to deal with stress through exercise, controlled breathing, meditation and techniques like yoga can help lower stress levels. Slow down if your pace of living has become too stressful.

Additional Heart-Healthy Suggestions

- **Stop smoking.** Smoking isn't just linked with lung disease. There is a link between smoking, high cholesterol and heart disease. Smoking can raise levels of LDL and accelerate atherosclerosis. Smoking can also lead to other heart problems. Since nicotine is a stimulant, cigarette smoke can cause blood vessels to constrict, meaning the heart has to work harder to pump blood. Smoking also increases the risk of blood clots.

- **Keep your weight at a healthy level.** Individuals with excess abdominal fat are at an increased risk of cardiovascular disease. Eat fruits and vegetables that are high in fiber and avoid the fatty foods discussed on page 28.
- **Reduce salt intake.** Salt intake is associated with obesity. And while sodium is a necessary nutrient, in excess it can be a cause of high blood pressure, another major risk factor in cardiovascular disease. Those with heart disease and high blood pressure should limit salt intake to 1500 mg per day.

Conclusion

Red yeast rice may be beneficial for those with moderately elevated cholesterol levels. Not only can red yeast rice lower cholesterol, but it is a natural compound with fewer potentially harmful side effects than prescription drugs. Combining red yeast rice therapy with dietary and lifestyle changes may contribute to better cardiovascular health.

References

Abd T.T., and T.A. Jacobson. "Statin-induced myopathy: a review and update." *Expert Opinion on Drug Safety*. Published electronically Feb. 23, 2011. doi 10.1517/14740338.2011.540568.

Ackermann R.T., C.D. Mulrow. et al. "Garlic shows promise for improving some cardiovascular risk factors." *Archives of Internal Medicine*. 161, no. 6 (March 2001): 813–24.

Akihisa T., H. Tokuda, et al. "Anti-tumor-initiating effects of monascin, an azaphilonoid pigment from the extract of Monascus pilosus fermented rice (red-mold rice)." *Chemistry and Biodiversity*. 2, no. 10 (Oct. 2005): 1305–9.

Alberts, A.W. "Discovery, Biochemistry and Biology of Lovastatin." *American Journal of Cardiology*. 62, no. 15 (Nov. 1988): 10J–15J.

Alizadeh-Navaei R., F., et al. "Investigation of the effect of ginger on the lipid levels. A double blind controlled clinical trial." *Saudi Medical Journal*. 29, no. 9 (Sept. 2008): 1280–4.

American Heart Association. "What Your Cholesterol Levels Mean." http://www.heart.org/HEARTORG/Conditions/Cholesterol/AboutCholesterol/What-Your-Cholesterol-Levels-Mean_UCM_305562_Article.jsp.

Bazzano L.A. "Effects of soluble dietary fiber on low-density lipoprotein cholesterol and coronary heart disease risk." *Current Atherosclerosis Reports*. 10, no. 6 (Dec. 2008): 473–7.

Becker, D.J. R.Y. Gordon, et al. "Red yeast rice for Dyslipidemia in Statin-Intolerant Patients: A Randomized Trial." *Annals of Internal Medicine*. 150, no. 12 (June 2009): 830–39.

Bliznakov, E.G. and D.J Wilkins. "Biochemical and Clinical Consequences of Inhibiting Coenzyme Q10 Biosynthesis by Lipid-Lowering HMG-CoA Reductase Inhibitors (Statins): A Critical Overview." *Advances in Therapy*. 15, no. 4 (July–Aug. 1998): 218–27.

Bokura, H. and S. Kobayashi. "Chitosan decreases total cholesterol in women: a randomized, double-blind, placebo-controlled trial." *European Journal of Clinical Nutrition*. 57, no. 5 (May 2003): 721–5.

Caso G., P. Kelly, et al. "Effect of coenzyme q10 on myopathic symptoms in patients treated with statins." *American Journal of Cardiology*. 99, no. 10 (May 2007): 1409–12.

Chen C.C., I.M. Liu. "Release of acetylcholine by Hon-Chi to raise insulin secretion in Wistar rats." *Neuroscience Letters.* 404, no. 1–2 (Aug. 2006): 117–21.

Endo, A, M. Kuroda, et al. "ML-235A, ML-236B, and ML-236C, new inhibitors of cholesterogenesis produced by penicillium citrinum." *Journal of Antibiotics.* 29 (1976): 1346–48.

Gordon R.Y., D.J. Becker. "The role of red yeast rice for the physician." *Current Atherosclerosis Report.* 13, no. 1 (Feb. 2011): 73–80.

Heber D., I. Yip, et al. "Cholesterol-lowering effects of a proprietary Chinese red-yeast-rice dietary supplement." *American Journal of Clinical Nutrition.* 69, no. 2 (Feb. 1999): 231–6.

Heber, D., A. Lembertas, et al. "An Analysis of Nine Proprietary Chinese Red Yeast Rice Dietary Supplements: Implications of Variability in Chemical Profile and Contents." *The Journal of Alternative and Complementary Medicine.* 7, no. 2 (2001): 133–9.

Hong M.Y., N.P. Seeram, et al. "Anticancer effects of Chinese red yeast rice versus monacolin K alone on colon cancer cells." *The Journal of Nutritional Biochemistry.* 19, no. 7 (July 2008): 448–58.

Hunninghake D.B., M.E. McGovern, et al. "A dose-ranging study of a new, once-daily, dual-component drug product containing niacin extended-release and lovastatin." *Clinical Cardiology.* 26, no. 3 (March 2003): 112–8.

Kris-Etherton P.M., W.S. Harris, et al. "Fish consumption, fish oil, omega-3 fatty acids, and cardiovascular disease." *Arteriosclerosis Thrombosis, and Vascular Biology.* 23, no. 2 (Feb. 2003): e20–30.

Kumar A., Kaur H., et al. "Role of coenzyme Q10 (CoQ10) in cardiac disease, hypertension and Meniere-like syndrome." *Pharmacology & Therapeutics.* 124, no. 3 (Dec. 2009): 259–68.

Lin W.Y., W.Y. Hsu, et al. "Proteome changes in Caco-2 cells treated with Monascus-fermented red mold rice extract." *Journal of Agricultural and Food Chemistry.* 55, no. 22 (Oct. 2007): 8987–94.

Liu L., S.P. Zhao SP, et al. "Xuezhikang decreases serum lipoprotein(a) and C-reactive protein concentrations in patients with coronary heart disease." *Clinical Chemistry.* 49, no. 8 (Aug. 2003): 1347–52.

Luepker, R.V. "Decline in Incident Coronary Heart Disease." *Circulation.* 117 (2008): 592–3.

Marschall H.U., C. Einarsson. "Gallstone disease." *Journal of Internal Medicine*. 261, no. 6 (June 2007): 529–42.

Mozaffarian D., R. Micha R, et al. "Effects on coronary heart disease of increasing polyunsaturated fat in place of saturated fat: a systematic review and meta-analysis of randomized controlled trials." *Public Library of Science Medicine*. Published electronically March 2010. doi: 10.1371/journal.pmed.1000252.

Natural Standard, s.v. "Coenzyme Q10." Accessed April 28, 2011. http://naturalstandard.com/databases/herbssupplement/coenzymeq10.asp.

Ostlund, R.E. Jr. "Phytosterols, cholesterol absorption and healthy diets." *Lipids*. 42, no. 1 (Feb. 2007): 41–5.

Singh B.B., S.P. Vinjamury, et al. "Ayurvedic and collateral herbal treatments for hyperlipidemia: a systematic review of randomized controlled trials and quasi-experimental designs." *Alternative Therapies in Health and Medicine*. 13, no. 4 (July–Aug. 2007): 22–8.

Spilburg C.A., Goldberg A.C., et al. "Fat-free foods supplemented with soy stanol-lecithin powder reduce cholesterol absorption and LDL cholesterol." *Journal of the American Dietetic Association*. 103, no. 5 (May 2003): 577–81.

Vacek J.L., G. Dittmeier, et al. "Comparison of lovastatin (20 mg) and nicotinic acid (1.2 g) with either drug alone for type II hyperlipoproteinemia." *American Journal of Cardiology*. 76, no. 3 (July 1995): 182–4.

Wang J., L. Zongliang L, et al. "Multicenter clinical trial of the serum lipid-lowering effects of a Monascus Purpureus (red yeast) rice preparation from traditional Chinese medicine." *Current Therapeutic Research*. 58, no. 12 (Dec. 1997): 964–78.

Yasukawa, K. M. Takahashi et al. "Inhibitory effect of oral administration of Monascus pigment on tumor production in two-stage carcinogenesis in mouse skin." *Oncology*. 53, no. 3 (May–June 1996): 247–9.

Zhao S.P., Z.L. Lu, et al. "Xuezhikang, an extract of cholestin, reduces cardiovascular events in type 2 diabetes patients with coronary heart disease: subgroup analysis of patients with type 2 diabetes from China coronary secondary prevention study (CCSPS)." *Journal of Cardiovascular Pharmacology*. 49, no. 2 (Feb. 2007): 81–4.